What is Yoga?

Yoga embraces several different disciplines, with the ultimate goal of unifying mind, body, and spirit with higher consciousness. Its origin lies in a system of Hindu Philosophy over 5,000 years old. The word yoga is derived from the Sanskrit "yuj" meaning "union."

What is the Yoga Book?

The Yoga Book is your personal yoga diary. It is used to record your thoughts and experiences in a yoga class. Often creative ideas, solutions to problems, and powerful insights are revealed to you - write them down! Included in the book is a glossary of different types of yoga. Enjoy!

Let the journey begin...

The journey of a thousand miles begins with one step. – Lao Tzu

Today's Date :

Style of Yoga/Type :

Notes/Thoughts : _____

_____

_____

_____

_____

_____

_____

_____

_____

_____

_____

_____

_____

_____

_____

_____

_____

_____

_____

_____

_____

_____

_____

_____

_____

Name of Instructor:

Wherever you go, go with all your heart. - Confucius

Today's Date :

Style of Yoga/Type :

Notes/Thoughts : _____

_____

_____

_____

_____

_____

_____

_____

_____

_____

_____

_____

_____

_____

_____

_____

_____

_____

_____

_____

_____

_____

_____

_____

_____

Name of Instructor:

Let the beauty of what you love be what you do. - Rumi

Today's Date :

Style of Yoga/Type :

Notes/Thoughts : _____

_____

_____

_____

_____

_____

_____

_____

_____

_____

_____

_____

_____

_____

_____

_____

_____

_____

_____

_____

_____

_____

_____

_____

Name of Instructor:

The greatness of a man's power is the measure of his surrender.
- William Booth

Today's Date :

Style of Yoga/Type :

Notes/Thoughts : _____

_____

_____

_____

_____

_____

_____

_____

_____

_____

_____

_____

_____

_____

_____

_____

_____

_____

_____

_____

_____

_____

Name of Instructor:

Everything in the universe is within you… - Rumi

Today's Date :

Style of Yoga/Type :

Notes/Thoughts : _____

_____

_____

_____

_____

_____

_____

_____

_____

_____

_____

_____

_____

_____

_____

_____

_____

_____

_____

_____

_____

_____

_____

_____

Name of Instructor:

I shut my eyes in order to see. - Paul Gauguin

Today's Date :

Style of Yoga/Type :

Notes/Thoughts : _____

_____

_____

_____

_____

_____

_____

_____

_____

_____

_____

_____

_____

_____

_____

_____

_____

_____

_____

_____

_____

_____

_____

Name of Instructor:

A loving heart is the truest wisdom. - Charles Dickens

Today's Date :

Style of Yoga/Type :

Notes/Thoughts : _____

_____

_____

_____

_____

_____

_____

_____

_____

_____

_____

_____

_____

_____

_____

_____

_____

_____

_____

_____

_____

_____

_____

_____

Name of Instructor:

Happiness is a perfume you cannot pour on others without
getting a few drops on yourself. - Ralph Waldo Emerson

Today's Date :

Style of Yoga/Type :

Notes/Thoughts : _____

_____

_____

_____

_____

_____

_____

_____

_____

_____

_____

_____

_____

_____

_____

_____

_____

_____

_____

_____

_____

_____

_____

Name of Instructor:

One can have no smaller or greater mastery than mastery
of oneself. - Leonardo da Vinci

Today's Date :

Style of Yoga/Type :

Notes/Thoughts : _____

_____

_____

_____

_____

_____

_____

_____

_____

_____

_____

_____

_____

_____

_____

_____

_____

_____

_____

_____

_____

_____

_____

Name of Instructor:

The power of imagination makes us infinite. – John Muir

Today's Date :

Style of Yoga/Type :

Notes/Thoughts : _____

_____

_____

_____

_____

_____

_____

_____

_____

_____

_____

_____

_____

_____

_____

_____

_____

_____

_____

_____

_____

_____

_____

_____

_____

Name of Instructor:

What you seek is seeking you. - Rumi

Today's Date :

Style of Yoga/Type :

Notes/Thoughts : _____

_____

_____

_____

_____

_____

_____

_____

_____

_____

_____

_____

_____

_____

_____

_____

_____

_____

_____

_____

_____

_____

_____

_____

_____

Name of Instructor:

To accomplish great things, we must dream as well as act.
- Anatole France

Today's Date :

Style of Yoga/Type :

Notes/Thoughts : _____

_____

_____

_____

_____

_____

_____

_____

_____

_____

_____

_____

_____

_____

_____

_____

_____

_____

_____

_____

_____

_____

Name of Instructor:

Knock on the sky and listen to the sound. - Zen Proverb

Today's Date :

Style of Yoga/Type :

Notes/Thoughts : _____

_____

_____

_____

_____

_____

_____

_____

_____

_____

_____

_____

_____

_____

_____

_____

_____

_____

_____

_____

_____

_____

_____

_____

Name of Instructor:

Be happy for this moment. This moment is your life.
- Omar Khayyam

Today's Date :

Style of Yoga/Type :

Notes/Thoughts : _____

_____

_____

_____

_____

_____

_____

_____

_____

_____

_____

_____

_____

_____

_____

_____

_____

_____

_____

_____

_____

_____

Name of Instructor:

Compassion is our deepest nature. It arises from our
interconnection with all things. - Buddhist Proverb

Today's Date :

Style of Yoga/Type :

Notes/Thoughts : _____

_____

_____

_____

_____

_____

_____

_____

_____

_____

_____

_____

_____

_____

_____

_____

_____

_____

_____

_____

_____

_____

_____

Name of Instructor:

A tranquil mind is not a little gift. - Sufi Proverb

Today's Date :

Style of Yoga/Type :

Notes/Thoughts : _____

_____

_____

_____

_____

_____

_____

_____

_____

_____

_____

_____

_____

_____

_____

_____

_____

_____

_____

_____

_____

_____

_____

_____

Name of Instructor:

Little by little, one walks far. – Peruvian Proverb

Today's Date :

Style of Yoga/Type :

Notes/Thoughts : _____

_____

_____

_____

_____

_____

_____

_____

_____

_____

_____

_____

_____

_____

_____

_____

_____

_____

_____

_____

_____

_____

Name of Instructor:

Nature does not hurry yet everything is accomplished.
- Taoist Proverb

Today's Date :

Style of Yoga/Type :

Notes/Thoughts : _____

_____

_____

_____

_____

_____

_____

_____

_____

_____

_____

_____

_____

_____

_____

_____

_____

_____

_____

_____

_____

_____

_____

Name of Instructor:

When fortune knocks upon the door, open it widely.
- Chilean Proverb

Today's Date :

Style of Yoga/Type :

Notes/Thoughts : _____

_____

_____

_____

_____

_____

_____

_____

_____

_____

_____

_____

_____

_____

_____

_____

_____

_____

_____

_____

_____

_____

_____

_____

_____

Name of Instructor:

In stillness the world is restored. – Buddhist Proverb

Today's Date :

Style of Yoga/Type :

Notes/Thoughts : _____

_____

_____

_____

_____

_____

_____

_____

_____

_____

_____

_____

_____

_____

_____

_____

_____

_____

_____

_____

_____

_____

_____

_____

_____

Name of Instructor:

From the withered tree, a flower blooms. - Zen Proverb

Today's Date :

Style of Yoga/Type :

Notes/Thoughts : _____

_____

_____

_____

_____

_____

_____

_____

_____

_____

_____

_____

_____

_____

_____

_____

_____

_____

_____

_____

_____

_____

_____

_____

_____

Name of Instructor:

The eye never forgets what the heart has seen. - African Proverb

Today's Date :

Style of Yoga/Type :

Notes/Thoughts : _____

_____

_____

_____

_____

_____

_____

_____

_____

_____

_____

_____

_____

_____

_____

_____

_____

_____

_____

_____

_____

_____

_____

_____

_____

_____

Name of Instructor:

And what he greatly thought, he nobly dared. - Homer

Today's Date :

Style of Yoga/Type :

Notes/Thoughts : _____

_____

_____

_____

_____

_____

_____

_____

_____

_____

_____

_____

_____

_____

_____

_____

_____

_____

_____

_____

_____

_____

_____

Name of Instructor:

The things we love tell us what we are. – St. Thomas Aquinas

Today's Date :

Style of Yoga/Type :

Notes/Thoughts : _____

_____

_____

_____

_____

_____

_____

_____

_____

_____

_____

_____

_____

_____

_____

_____

_____

_____

_____

_____

_____

_____

Name of Instructor:

The obstacle is the path. - Zen Proverb

Today's Date :

Style of Yoga/Type :

Notes/Thoughts : _____

_____

_____

_____

_____

_____

_____

_____

_____

_____

_____

_____

_____

_____

_____

_____

_____

_____

_____

_____

_____

_____

_____

_____

_____

_____

_____

Name of Instructor:

Freedom is the right to live as we wish. – Epictetus

Today's Date :

Style of Yoga/Type :

Notes/Thoughts : _____

_____

_____

_____

_____

_____

_____

_____

_____

_____

_____

_____

_____

_____

_____

_____

_____

_____

_____

_____

_____

_____

_____

_____

_____

_____

Name of Instructor:

Music in the soul can be heard by the universe. - Taoist Proverb

Today's Date :

Style of Yoga/Type :

Notes/Thoughts : _____

_____

_____

_____

_____

_____

_____

_____

_____

_____

_____

_____

_____

_____

_____

_____

_____

_____

_____

_____

_____

_____

_____

_____

Name of Instructor:

Experience this moment to its fullest. - Zen Proverb

Today's Date :

Style of Yoga/Type :

Notes/Thoughts : _____

_____

_____

_____

_____

_____

_____

_____

_____

_____

_____

_____

_____

_____

_____

_____

_____

_____

_____

_____

_____

_____

_____

_____

Name of Instructor:

Do what is right, come what may. - Spanish Proverb

Today's Date :

Style of Yoga/Type :

Notes/Thoughts : _____

_____

_____

_____

_____

_____

_____

_____

_____

_____

_____

_____

_____

_____

_____

_____

_____

_____

_____

_____

_____

_____

_____

_____

Name of Instructor:

You yourself, as much as anybody in the entire universe,
deserve your love and attention. - Buddha

Today's Date :

Style of Yoga/Type :

Notes/Thoughts : _____

_____

_____

_____

_____

_____

_____

_____

_____

_____

_____

_____

_____

_____

_____

_____

_____

_____

_____

_____

_____

_____

_____

_____

_____

Name of Instructor:

Give light and the darkness will disappear… - Desiderius Erasmus

Today's Date :

Style of Yoga/Type :

Notes/Thoughts : _____

_____

_____

_____

_____

_____

_____

_____

_____

_____

_____

_____

_____

_____

_____

_____

_____

_____

_____

_____

_____

_____

_____

Name of Instructor:

There is nothing stronger in the world than gentleness. - Han Syin

Today's Date :

Style of Yoga/Type :

Notes/Thoughts : _____

_____

_____

_____

_____

_____

_____

_____

_____

_____

_____

_____

_____

_____

_____

_____

_____

_____

_____

_____

_____

_____

Name of Instructor:

Even if I knew that tomorrow the world would go to pieces,
I would still plant my apple tree. – Martin Luther

Today's Date :

Style of Yoga/Type :

Notes/Thoughts : _____

_____

_____

_____

_____

_____

_____

_____

_____

_____

_____

_____

_____

_____

_____

_____

_____

_____

_____

_____

_____

_____

_____

Name of Instructor:

The glow of one warm thought is to me worth more than money. - Thomas Jefferson

Today's Date :

Style of Yoga/Type :

Notes/Thoughts : _____

_____

_____

_____

_____

_____

_____

_____

_____

_____

_____

_____

_____

_____

_____

_____

_____

_____

_____

_____

_____

_____

_____

_____

Name of Instructor:

What we achieve inwardly will change outer reality. - Plutarch

Today's Date :

Style of Yoga/Type :

Notes/Thoughts : _____

_____

_____

_____

_____

_____

_____

_____

_____

_____

_____

_____

_____

_____

_____

_____

_____

_____

_____

_____

_____

_____

_____

_____

_____

Name of Instructor:

When the heart is full the tongue will speak. - Scottish Proverb

Today's Date :

Style of Yoga/Type :

Notes/Thoughts : _____

_____

_____

_____

_____

_____

_____

_____

_____

_____

_____

_____

_____

_____

_____

_____

_____

_____

_____

_____

_____

_____

_____

_____

_____

Name of Instructor:

Patience is the companion of wisdom. - Saint Augustine

Today's Date :

Style of Yoga/Type :

Notes/Thoughts : _____

_____

_____

_____

_____

_____

_____

_____

_____

_____

_____

_____

_____

_____

_____

_____

_____

_____

_____

_____

_____

_____

_____

_____

_____

Name of Instructor:

Fill the rest of your life with your dreams and live the
unforgettable. - Fyodor Doetovsky

Today's Date :

Style of Yoga/Type :

Notes/Thoughts : _____

_____

_____

_____

_____

_____

_____

_____

_____

_____

_____

_____

_____

_____

_____

_____

_____

_____

_____

_____

_____

_____

_____

_____

_____

Name of Instructor:

Believe you can and you're halfway there. – Theodore Roosevelt

Today's Date :

Style of Yoga/Type :

Notes/Thoughts : _____

_____

_____

_____

_____

_____

_____

_____

_____

_____

_____

_____

_____

_____

_____

_____

_____

_____

_____

_____

_____

_____

_____

_____

Name of Instructor:

Love gives life within. – Hawaiin Proverb

Today's Date :

Style of Yoga/Type :

Notes/Thoughts : _____

_____

_____

_____

_____

_____

_____

_____

_____

_____

_____

_____

_____

_____

_____

_____

_____

_____

_____

_____

_____

_____

_____

Name of Instructor:

Be yourself; everyone else is already taken. - Oscar Wilde

Today's Date :

Style of Yoga/Type :

Notes/Thoughts : _____

_____

_____

_____

_____

_____

_____

_____

_____

_____

_____

_____

_____

_____

_____

_____

_____

_____

_____

_____

_____

_____

_____

_____

_____

Name of Instructor:

Our truest life is when we are in dreams awake.
- Henry David Thoreau

Today's Date :

Style of Yoga/Type :

Notes/Thoughts : _____

_____

_____

_____

_____

_____

_____

_____

_____

_____

_____

_____

_____

_____

_____

_____

_____

_____

_____

_____

_____

_____

_____

_____

_____

Name of Instructor:

It is always the simple that produces the marvelous. - Amelia Barr

Today's Date :

Style of Yoga/Type :

Notes/Thoughts : _____

_____

_____

_____

_____

_____

_____

_____

_____

_____

_____

_____

_____

_____

_____

_____

_____

_____

_____

_____

_____

_____

_____

_____

_____

Name of Instructor:

No man ever steps in the same river twice, for it's not the
same river and he's not the same man. – Heraclitus

Today's Date :

Style of Yoga/Type :

Notes/Thoughts : _____

_____

_____

_____

_____

_____

_____

_____

_____

_____

_____

_____

_____

_____

_____

_____

_____

_____

_____

_____

_____

_____

_____

Name of Instructor:

In a place where there is will, there is a road. - Korean Proverb

Today's Date :

Style of Yoga/Type :

Notes/Thoughts : _____

_____

_____

_____

_____

_____

_____

_____

_____

_____

_____

_____

_____

_____

_____

_____

_____

_____

_____

_____

_____

Name of Instructor:

An effort made for the happiness of others lifts us above
ourselves. - Lydia M. Child

Today's Date :

Style of Yoga/Type :

Notes/Thoughts : _____

_____

_____

_____

_____

_____

_____

_____

_____

_____

_____

_____

_____

_____

_____

_____

_____

_____

_____

_____

_____

_____

_____

Name of Instructor:

For after all, the best thing one can do when it is raining is
let it rain. - Henry Wadsworth Longfellow

Today's Date :

Style of Yoga/Type :

Notes/Thoughts : _____

_____

_____

_____

_____

_____

_____

_____

_____

_____

_____

_____

_____

_____

_____

_____

_____

_____

_____

_____

_____

_____

_____

_____

_____

Name of Instructor:

Love in its essence is spiritual fire. - Lucius Annaeus Seneca

Today's Date :

Style of Yoga/Type :

Notes/Thoughts : _____

_____

_____

_____

_____

_____

_____

_____

_____

_____

_____

_____

_____

_____

_____

_____

_____

_____

_____

_____

_____

_____

Name of Instructor:

Much wisdom often goes with fewer words. - Sophocles

Today's Date :

Style of Yoga/Type :

Notes/Thoughts : _____

_____

_____

_____

_____

_____

_____

_____

_____

_____

_____

_____

_____

_____

_____

_____

_____

_____

_____

_____

_____

_____

_____

_____

_____

Name of Instructor:

Fear less, hope more; whine less, breathe more; talk less, say more;
hate less, love more; and all good things are yours. – Swedish Proverb

Today's Date :

Style of Yoga/Type :

Notes/Thoughts : _____

_____

_____

_____

_____

_____

_____

_____

_____

_____

_____

_____

_____

_____

_____

_____

_____

_____

_____

_____

_____

_____

_____

Name of Instructor:

Fall seven times and stand up eight. - Japanese Proverb

Today's Date :

Style of Yoga/Type :

Notes/Thoughts : _____

_____

_____

_____

_____

_____

_____

_____

_____

_____

_____

_____

_____

_____

_____

_____

_____

_____

_____

_____

_____

_____

_____

Name of Instructor:

The trees that are slow to grow bear the best fruit. – Moliere

Today's Date :

Style of Yoga/Type :

Notes/Thoughts : _____

_____

_____

_____

_____

_____

_____

_____

_____

_____

_____

_____

_____

_____

_____

_____

_____

_____

_____

_____

_____

_____

_____

_____

_____

Name of Instructor:

If not us, who? If not now, when? - Hillel the Elder

Today's Date :

Style of Yoga/Type :

Notes/Thoughts : _____

_____

_____

_____

_____

_____

_____

_____

_____

_____

_____

_____

_____

_____

_____

_____

_____

_____

_____

_____

_____

_____

_____

_____

Name of Instructor:

Let a hundred flowers bloom, let a hundred schools of
thought contend. - Mao Zedong

Today's Date :

Style of Yoga/Type :

Notes/Thoughts : _____

_____

_____

_____

_____

_____

_____

_____

_____

_____

_____

_____

_____

_____

_____

_____

_____

_____

_____

_____

_____

_____

_____

Name of Instructor:

The real voyage of discovery consists not of seeking new landscapes, but in having new eyes. - Marcel Proust

Today's Date :

Style of Yoga/Type :

Notes/Thoughts : _____

_____

_____

_____

_____

_____

_____

_____

_____

_____

_____

_____

_____

_____

_____

_____

_____

_____

_____

_____

_____

_____

_____

_____

_____

Name of Instructor:

Certain things catch your eye, but pursue only those that
capture the heart. - Native American Proverb

Today's Date :

Style of Yoga/Type :

Notes/Thoughts : _____

_____

_____

_____

_____

_____

_____

_____

_____

_____

_____

_____

_____

_____

_____

_____

_____

_____

_____

_____

_____

_____

_____

_____

_____

Name of Instructor:

Virtue is bold, and goodness never fearful. – William Shakespeare

Today's Date :

Style of Yoga/Type :

Notes/Thoughts : _____

_____

_____

_____

_____

_____

_____

_____

_____

_____

_____

_____

_____

_____

_____

_____

_____

_____

_____

_____

_____

_____

_____

Name of Instructor:

The two most important days in your life are the day you
are born and the day you find out why. - Mark Twain

Today's Date :

Style of Yoga/Type :

Notes/Thoughts : _____

_____

_____

_____

_____

_____

_____

_____

_____

_____

_____

_____

_____

_____

_____

_____

_____

_____

_____

_____

_____

_____

_____

_____

_____

Name of Instructor:

Experience is the teacher of all things. - Julius Caesar

Today's Date :

Style of Yoga/Type :

Notes/Thoughts : _____

_____

_____

_____

_____

_____

_____

_____

_____

_____

_____

_____

_____

_____

_____

_____

_____

_____

_____

_____

_____

_____

Name of Instructor:

It is no use waiting for your ship to come in unless you have sent one out. – Belgian Proverb

Today's Date :

Style of Yoga/Type :

Notes/Thoughts : _____

_____

_____

_____

_____

_____

_____

_____

_____

_____

_____

_____

_____

_____

_____

_____

_____

_____

_____

_____

_____

_____

_____

_____

_____

Name of Instructor:

Yoga Glossary

Bhakti-yoga: 'Yoga of Devotion' *A Classic Yoga*
A practice of devotion and concentration on a higher consciousness.

Hatha-yoga: 'Yoga of Physical Movement' *A Classic Yoga*
A practice of poses, postures, and breathing. It is the yoga of physical movement and the most commonly known yoga in the world.

*There are several different styles of Hatha-yoga. Students are encouraged to research these different types, try different styles, and note their experiences, in an attempt to determine which style is right for the student.

Jnana-yoga: 'Yoga of Enlightenment' *A Classic Yoga*
The path of wisdom and inner knowingness.

Karma-yoga: 'Yoga of Right Actions' *A Classic Yoga*
A practice of doing everything, everyday with the mind centered on a higher consciousness.

Raja-yoga: 'Yoga of Meditation' *A Classic Yoga*
A practice of exercise, breathing, meditation, and learning.

The Yoga Book does not accept responsibility for anything resulting from the practice of yoga; including any consequence, injury, result, or effect on the body, etc. so please consult a physician before engaging in the practice of yoga.